Shingles Relief

Shingles Relief

How to Relieve the Pain Of Herpes Zoster, Treat the Herpes Virus, And Prevent Future Outbreaks

Deborah Bleecker, LAc, MSOM

Disclaimer

This book contains the opinions and ideas of the author. It is intended to provide helpful and informative material on the subjects addressed. It is sold with the understanding that the author and publisher are not engaged in rendering medical, health, psychological or any other type of advice or services in the book. If the reader needs personal, medical, health, or other assistance or advice, a competent professional should be consulted.

The author and publisher disclaim any responsibility for any liability, loss or risk, either personal or otherwise that occurs as a consequence, directly or indirectly, of the use and application of the contents of this book.

ISBN 978-1-940146-79-9
Library of Congress Control Number 2018905745
Draycott Publishing, LLC

Contents

Introduction

If you are reading this introduction, you or someone you know probably has shingles. You are desperately looking for answers to how to help yourself or your loved one. You might have already seen medical doctors and taken all the medications you were prescribed, yet you still have pain.

I was in the same position. Although I am an acupuncturist, with over 20 years of successfully treating diseases like migraine headaches, anxiety, any type of pain, insomnia, fatigue, digestive problems, autoimmune diseases, and just about any disorder you can think of, I did not know how to treat shingles.

My mom is 79 years old and she got shingles. The pain was so horrific that she could not sleep at night. Touching the lesions with even something as light as a cotton shirt was agonizing for her. The pain was described as a burning, stabbing, and shooting pain. Even when she sat still, she had pain from her spine to her abdomen.

I was desperate for answers, because some of the most common treatments, including acupuncture, were not working on her. The antiviral drugs did not work, the pain pills did not work. Nothing was working. I had to find answers. Many people suffer from horrible residual pain from shingles. They can have it for many years. That is especially common in people over 60.

After much research, I discovered which techniques work best to relieve shingles pain fast. I have also learned which herbs and herbal formulas are most effective, in addition to which vitamins are best to treat the virus, and heal the nerve damage that shingles causes.

In my experience as an acupuncturist, there is almost always a way to resolve health problems. You just have to not give up, and to keep looking for answers. Do not accept defeat. There is always an answer.

This book is a shortcut to the remedies and techniques that work the best for shingles. There are many treatment options that work. You just choose the one you prefer and start. I have included the brand names and exact supplements that were tried, so you will not waste money on supplements that are not as effective.

Herpes Virus Treatment

If you are looking for effective remedies to prevent and treat any type of herpes, including genital herpes, the herbal formulas in this book will work. I have had patients who kept a supply of the herbal formula I recommend for shingles. They take it at the first sign of an outbreak, and it usually subsides quickly. I would also recommend the immune tonics in the chapter on preventing future outbreaks.

Chapter 1

Hospital Treatment and Warnings for Caregivers

Shingles can cause such pain and nausea that you might need to go to the hospital. I wanted to recount my experiences there, because it gives you a good idea of how contagious shingles is and how they treat it in the hospital.

My mom went to the hospital because the shingles virus affected her stomach, and she could not keep down food or water. She had to be rehydrated at the hospital. If you have nausea or vomiting, please consider seeking professional medical help. You can die from dehydration. The staff at the hospital will be able to give you intravenous fluids to restore your mineral levels. You can easily become deficient in potassium and magnesium.

In the emergency room, they gave her antiviral drugs, morphine for pain, and rehydration liquids. She stayed in the hospital for several days. The reason I am telling you about this is that she was put in isolation. She was put in a room and the staff entered via a negative pressure room. They entered her room via a separate room, put on a new paper gown, and gloves, every time they went into her room.

Shingles is Contagious

The staff would not touch her without wearing gloves, and they were not allowed to touch things that she had touched. No one could enter via the main door, because the virus was shedding, so the other people at the hospital could be affected. She said they made her feel like an outcast, but this was necessary to protect everyone.

Although some people say that you cannot catch the shingles, if you have not had the chickenpox, you might get infected. Even if you had the chickenpox, this is a horrible virus, and it can affect your immune system. During the first month of my mom's shingles, I felt like I had the flu. When you are around a person with shingles, you can easily breathe in viral particles, and they can affect caregivers. I took Chinese herbs like Long Dan Xie Gan Tang, and Zhong Gan Ling, which treat viruses very well. Long Dan Xie Gan Tang is explained in the Antiviral supplement chapter. It treats all types of herpes viruses. If you can take it in the beginning of the outbreak, you might be able to stop it in its tracks.

Do Not Touch Shingles Lesions

No one should touch the shingles lesions without washing their hands afterwards. There is chance that the shingles could spread to other parts of the body. People can get shingles on any part of their body. Shingles of the eye occurs when the nerve root that is associated with the eye is affected. Shingles can cause blindness. Seek medical help immediately. Continue seeking help, and see your eye doctor if your eye is affected.

Clothing and sheets should be washed daily. The virus sheds everywhere the patient goes, and those viral particles will stay where they are dropped until they are removed. The shingles lesions ooze, and the affected area will shed for weeks. They say that once the lesions have crusted over, they are no longer dangerous to other people. I personally do not want to take that risk. If you are anywhere near someone with shingles, do not touch them or touch things they have touched.

They gave her blood thinner drugs, because sitting all day can make you more prone to have a blood clot. The morphine did not help much to relieve the pain.

Chickenpox and Shingles are Contagious

If you are exposed to someone who has the shingles and you have not had chickenpox, you can contract chickenpox. It is the same virus. If you have had chickenpox and are around someone with shingles, you could get shingles, because the virus is already in your body.

Being around someone who has the active shingles virus outbreak can mean that your shingles breaks out. The virus is lurking in your body, waiting for its chance to take over. If you take care of yourself, by taking the supplements in the antiviral chapter, and the "prevent future shingles" chapter, you might actually reduce the chance that you get shingles yourself. People who are repeatedly exposed to the virus are building up immunity to the disease.

If I had known then what I know now, I would have used wet cupping as soon as we knew it was shingles. I think it is the least painful therapy, and most effective thing to do for shingles. Please refer to the cupping chapter to learn about that.

SHINGLES RELIEF

Chapter 2

Shingles Symptoms and Dermatome Maps

If you can catch your shingles in the early stage, it is much easier to treat. You will often not know that it is shingles until the rash erupts. It can start in any location.

The most common symptoms of shingles are:

- Pain, burning, numbness or tingling.
- Sensitivity to even light touch.
- A red rash that begins a few days after the first signs of pain.
- Fluid-filled blisters that break open, and eventually crust over.
- Itching.

Itching tingling and pain are the first symptoms. The location of the pain is determined by which nerve root is affected. The herpes virus settles into the spinal nerves and once it is reactivated, it spreads from the spine to the front of the abdomen, or to any other location on the body. The affected nerve usually stops at the midline, which is the middle of your abdomen.

Dermatomes

The pain usually affects the whole nerve, starting at the spine. It radiates down the nerve dermatomes. This shows you the path of the pain. The virus attacks the entire nerve. It only surfaces at various locations, but it is still affecting the nerve inside.

You can see from the Dermatome images that each spinal nerve is associated with a vertebrae. C is cervical, or neck. If these nerves are affected, you can get shingles on your face. T, or TH in one of the images, stands for thoracic. This is the upper back. L is lumbar, or lower back. S is sacrum, or tailbone. It is not known why shingles affects a particular nerve. Some people get it on the face, some the upper back, and some the lower back, or legs.

Dermatomes

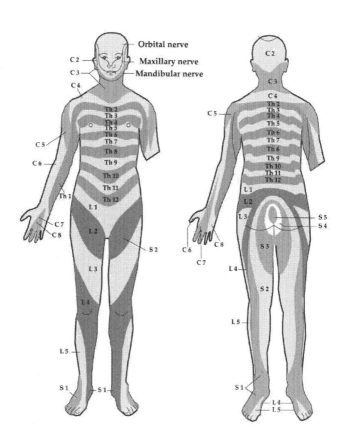

Dermatomes

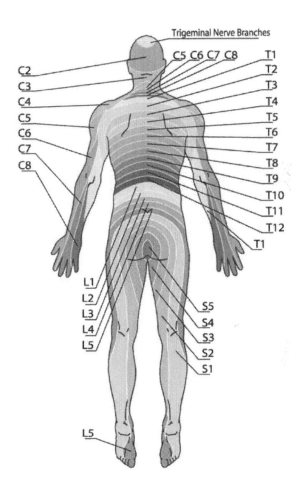

Trigeminal Nerve Branches

C5 C6 C7 C8

C2
C3
C4
C5
C6
C7
C8

T1
T2
T3
T4
T5
T6
T7
T8
T9
T10
T11
T12
T1

L1
L2
L3
L4
L5

S5
S4
S3
S2
S1

L5

In Chinese medicine, shingles is likened to a snake. It has a head and a tail. Some people describe the sensation as a snake moving around inside. After I did wet cupping, that evening the sensation of the snake moving around increased. I believe that is the body fighting off the virus.

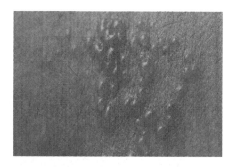

Common symptoms are chills, fever, and body aches, with pain in the affected areas. When the virus reaches the skin, you will feel a tingly sensation, with slight burning. When the lesion erupts, you will see the fluid filled blister with red rings around it. The blister has active virus particles in it. You should be very careful to not touch the lesions with your bare hands before touching another part of your body, because the virus can be spread by doing this.

Sharp shooting pains every few minutes can last the duration of the shingles, and if not resolved completely, the nerves can be affected and cause pain for years. This is caused post herpetic neuralgia. It is my belief that some residual nerve pain might be caused by an active virus. The virus has to be subdued by the immune system to make it go dormant again. It was dormant before you had the current outbreak. But your immune system has to be strong enough to make this happen. That is where the anti-viral supplements, and other therapies come into play.

The skin is very sensitive to the touch. The sufferer cannot be touched, and cannot have clothing or sheets sitting on top of the skin. The skin is hypersensitive.

Shingles is caused by a virus. When your body fights off a virus, you might have other viral symptoms. Digestion is often affected, which can cause nausea, and vomiting. It can also make it harder to digest meals.

Fatigue is common with shingles. It is very helpful if you can take herbal supplements to boost your immune system, and your energy in general. Having a virus, and being in severe pain will quickly sap your energy levels. The herbs in the chapter on preventing future shingles attacks will improve your health.

Chapter 3

Topical Pain Relievers

Topical pain relievers are great, because they often work faster than internal products. Applying the product topically means you often need less of the active pain relieving ingredient, so you are less likely to be affected negatively internally. Aspirin and other medications can damage your intestines if they are taken too long, or on an empty stomach. They are not designed to be used long term.

Patch Test All Topical Products

All the topical pain relievers work temporarily. They might cause skin irritation on shingles lesions. I think it is important to resolve the shingles virus by taking anti-viral supplements, and doing therapies like plum blossom therapy, and cupping therapy, but these products did work to relieve pain. Please be sure to patch test anything you use topically. Apply it to a small area first, to see how your skin reacts.

When looking for shingles pain relief, you will find a lot of products that claim to relieve shingles pain. I am including information on which supplements worked for us, and a few that did not work, as a reference. Please remember that all products, both internal and external, will work differently for different people. You might get great results with things that did not work for us.

We found that the pain relief was temporary. It would usually last about 6 hours, then it irritated the skin. Some creams, like Manuka cream, did not work at all. That is supposed to be anti-viral, because it contains Manuka honey. Some recommend smearing Manuka honey all over your lesions. I think the anti-virals do not penetrate the skin enough to be effective for most people. We even tried olive leaf extract oil. It did nothing. That is a strong anti-viral that can be taken internally for many types of viruses.

Six Week Trials

There are a lot of articles online about topical shingles pain relievers. The problem with a lot of them is that they do a trial of the product for six weeks, to determine how effective the product is. Since most shingles pain is resolved within that time period with no interventions, I don't think a six week trial is meaningful. I want immediate pain relief. So bear that in mind if you do further research online for solutions.

Capsaicin Cream, or Cayenne Cream

Some people suggest Capsaicin cream for pain relief. I do not really recommend this. The idea behind this is that the cream will reduce the pain over time. Most research I have found on this is quoted at a six week timeframe for it to be effective. In the meantime, you are rubbing hot pepper on your skin, when it is already very sensitive. Many people have a resolution of their pain after six weeks anyway. That is if they are healthy enough to overcome the virus on their own. I would not wait six weeks for relief. Capsaicin is derived from hot peppers. Some medical doctors prescribe this.

Essential Oils

Essential oils are the concentrated extracts of plants, often flowers. There are several essential oils that can be used to relieve shingles pain. The oil we found most effective was St. John's Wort. We used the Herb Pharm brand. This herb is usually prescribed to relieve depression. It can also be used internally as a nervine. The results were temporary, but it was effective for about six hours.

St. John's Wort oil can be used internally for the virus, although I do not believe it is the strongest anti-viral herb available. It works very well externally to relieve the pain.

Geranium oil is an effective option for pain relief. This oil can be applied at full strength, or mixed with a carrier oil, such as grape seed oil. One reference I found said that using it full strength was reported to be more effective than diluting it. Most essential oils need to be diluted to use on the skin. I would experiment and see which one works best for you, if you try it. It has a nice smell, although pungent. It is also relaxing.

Clove oil is used by dentists to treat dry sockets. It is a natural anti-bacterial and numbing agent. This oil was in the wood lock oil we used that was so effective. It ended up irritating her skin after about eight hours. But it was the first oil to give her relief.

Black cumin seed oil is recommended by some sources. We did not find it effective at all. It is also called black seed oil.

Peppermint oil is an ingredient in many topical pain relievers. In one case, a woman with post herpetic neuralgia used pure peppermint oil to relieve pain. The name of the article is "A novel treatment of postherpetic neuralgia using peppermint oil." It stated that during the two months of her treatment she had minor side effects, yet the peppermint oil continued to relieve her pain. We did not try this oil. I believe this woman would have benefited from anti-viral vitamins and herbs, rather than masking the pain with a topical pain reliever long-term.

Terrasil Shingles Skincare Ointment

This is a cream that contains zinc, which helps slow down viral replication, peppermint oil, which is a pain reliever, and bentonite clay. We did not try this ointment, but I wanted to mention it, because I read that zinc ointment was helpful. This is sold at drug stores.

Natural Moisturizer

Shingles makes it harder to keep your skin moist, because so many things irritate it. My mom found Alba Botanica lotions to be very soothing. They are made with natural oils, and contain no mineral oil or petrolatum. Whatever you put on your skin is usually absorbed into your body. Some people say you should not put it on your skin if you would not be willing to eat it.

Alba Botanica carries several types of lotion. The best option for sensitive skin is Very Emollient Lotion, Original. After your shingles are over, you can try their Maximum formula. It has glycolic acid in it, which helps to exfoliate dead skin. I would not put it on shingles affected skin.

Apple Cider Vinegar

This relieved pain almost immediately. You can just dab it on with a cotton ball. Some sources say to dilute it. When it dries out, it tends to irritate the skin. Vinegar is acidic. In my experience, this does work temporarily.

Willow Balm

This product has willow bark extract in it. Aspirin used to be derived from willow bark, which is a natural pain reliever. Instead of taking aspirin, you can try using willow bark extract. When you use an herb in its natural state, you are less likely to have negative side effects. When a component of an herb is isolated, such as making aspirin out of willow bark, you remove the other components that actually balance the herb and make it less likely to cause side effects.

Willow Balm ingredients are: Water, Mineral Oil, Lipowax D/Hallstar NCD-20, Lipo GMS 470, Cetyl Alcohol, Stearic Acid, Stearyl Alcohol, Propylene Glycol, Isopropyl Palmitate, Sweet Almond Oil, Jojoba Oil, Optiphen Plus, Menthol, Camphor, White Willow Bark, Geranium Bourbon, Lavender 40/42, Spearmint,

Helichrysum gymnocephalum, Eucalyptus Globulus. It has menthol at a level of 3%. If you notice, it has menthol and camphor, which are topical pain relievers in many products. It includes geranium oil, which is helpful for shingles, as well as Spearmint, which is an effective topical pain reliever.

Wood Lock Oil

Wood lock oil is the first topical pain reliever we tried. This was the first supplement that relieved pain. The version we used had clove oil in it. This product is a traditional Chinese remedy that is useful for many problems. It is great for back and neck pain. You can also use a tiny amount near the sinuses to relieve sinus congestion.

The problem with wood lock oil, is that the ingredients might be too strong to use regularly on shingles skin. It has alcohol in high levels. It has methyl salicylate in it, which is similar to a topical aspirin. The brand you will find easily is the Wong To Yick brand from Hong Kong. The ingredients are: Menthol 16.49g Methyl salicylate 14.55g Camphor 4.36g. You might not find this product irritating. I would only consider applying it once a day.

Best Results for Topical Pain Reliever

My first choice for topical pain relievers would be St. John's Wort oil. It was the most effective at relieving pain. I would consider diluting it with grape seed oil for topical application. I believe Willow Balm is a good option also.

I would recommend not using any topical pain relievers if you are on blood thinners. Please consult your healthcare provider on this. All products applied on the skin can be absorbed internally. You should also patch test your skin. Do not apply any product on all of your lesions without trying it on a small area first. That is important advice for any topical product. Everyone reacts differently to products.

SHINGLES RELIEF

Chapter 4

Anti-Viral Herbs and Supplements

There are hundreds of herbs that can be used to treat viruses. Some herbs are effective to treat certain types of viruses, but are not as effective on treat others. This chapter is a quick survey of the best antiviral supplements I found that are effective against shingles.

What Not To Eat

Before I explain what supplements can be used to treat viruses, I want to make sure you know that certain foods provide higher levels of the amino acid arginine. This can make the herpes virus worse. These food include chocolate, nuts, seeds, beans, and soy. I would avoid these foods as much as possible for best results. Peanuts are included. They are technically beans, not nuts.

To treat shingles, supplements that boost the immune system, and kill the virus at the same time, are a good option. There are many supplements that treat viruses. They type of virus you are treating determines which herb will work the best.

Vitamin C in High Doses

One source suggests 2,000 mg of vitamin C every hour. This is called bowel tolerance. Your body will continue to absorb vitamin C to fight the virus. Once you have taken too much, you will have loose stools. Reduce your dosage to just below that level and take for three days minimum.

Since it is so difficult for most people to find someone who will do vitamin C injections, an easier option is to take high doses of vitamin C. I also like liposomal vitamin C. This is absorbed much better than regular vitamin C. Dr. Thomas E. Levy has a great website with a lot of articles on how vitamin C works to treat many ailments.

Your body uses vitamin C to kill viruses. I had whooping cough several years ago. I tried every anti-viral and anti-bacterial herb I knew, nothing worked. After spending three months with this disease, I found research online that vitamin C would resolve it. It worked. I took 8,000 mg a day for a few days until the cough was gone.

I think we have only scraped the surface of what vitamin C can do for us. The main reason people do not get results is they do not take enough. Most people are already deficient in vitamin C, so when they get sick, they need even more to treat the disease.

There are reports of very high doses of vitamin C resolving shingles pain entirely. When you are already sick, it can be hard to take high doses of anything. Having shingles is like having a combination of the flu, which is also viral, and the worst pain you have ever had. Often the stomach is unsettled, or the person is nauseated for days. It is not uncommon for it to cause nausea and vomiting, which makes it difficult to take supplements.

Emergen-C Powder, Vitamin C Supplement

If you do not want to take a lot of pills, Emergen C makes a great vitamin C powder. You can choose which flavor you prefer. They currently have cherry, raspberry, orange, blueberry-acai, acai, tropical, tangerine, cranberry-pomegranate, and citrus flavors.

Liposomal Vitamin C from LivonLabs

This vitamin C is much better absorbed than regular ascorbic acid vitamin C. Here is a quote from their website, "LivOnLabs' patented Lypo-Spheric™ Vitamin C encapsulates the C molecules in liposomes made from Essential Phospholipids." If you decide to try this type of vitamin C, you might also find a product by Dr. Mercola. I believe this is not the same product as in the LivonLabs brand. Their website is at www.livonlabs.com.

This type of vitamin C is optional. It is in a gel form, and must be mixed with liquid. Take the type of vitamin C you prefer.

B Vitamins

All B vitamins are helpful for nerve issues. Many people are deficient in these vitamins and have nerve issues as a result. B 12 is particularly helpful for nerve pain. Taking a B complex vitamin like the Raw series from the Garden of Life is a good option.

L Lysine

Lysine is an amino acid that is very popular to prevent and treat herpes simplex. People who get fever blisters use this at the first sign of an outbreak, and can often prevent it from being a full blown outbreak. A common dosage is 1,000 to 1,500 mg four times a day. It inhibits the herpes virus from reproducing.

Vitamin E

The dosage for vitamin E is 400 to 800 IU daily. I like Jarrow Famil-E. Solgar also makes a good product. It is mixed tocopherols. There are different kinds of vitamin E, it is good to take a blend, if you can.

Zinc

Zinc is effective to reduce how much the virus can replicate itself. It is popular in natural cough drops for example. When you have a cold or flu, the virus spreads to your lungs via your throat. If you take zinc lozenges, it will reduce the likelihood of a lung infection. The recommended dosage is 15-20 mg of zinc every three hours, for up to three days. Do not take too much zinc. Nature's Way makes a berry flavor lozenge. The label says to not exceed 6 lozenges per day, and to not take it for more than a week.

Olive Leaf Extract

This is a very effective anti-viral, and anti-toxin. It is the first choice for single herbs used to treat viruses. It is important to take the extract of the herb, not the raw herb. An extract is made by boiling the herbs, and making a concentrated product from that. It is more easily absorbed, and you can take fewer pills. I like the Nature's Way brand.

Long Dan Xie Gan Tang

This is one of the most effective Chinese herbal formulas to relieve herpes. It is very effective to prevent and treat genital and oral herpes. It is also shown to be effective against shingles. It is used for many things in Chinese medicine. It treats acid reflux, and severe stress.

People who suffer from genital and oral herpes can take this at the first sign of a breakout. If you catch it early, you might easily prevent a full blown breakout.

Viola Clear Fire

A Chinese herbal formula that is useful for any type of herpes is Viola Clear Fire, by Golden Flower Chinese herbs. The Chinese name for this formula is Di Ding Qing Huo Pain. I know you probably did not want to know the Chinese name, but your acupuncturist will.

The types of viral problems that this formula addresses are chickenpox, genital sores, any type of herpes, laryngitis, mononucleosis, sinus infection, and tonsillitis, to name a few. These antiviral herbs are:

Hedyotis Oldenlandia, Bai Hua She She Cao
Houttuynia, Yu Xing Cao
Viola, Zi Hua Di Ding
Isatis Leaf, Da Qing Ye
Isatis Root, Ban Lan Gen
Andrographis, Chuan Xin Lian
Japanese Honeysuckle Flower, Jin Yin Hua

Self-Heal Spike, Xia Ku Cao
Forsythia Fruit, Lian Qiao
Tangerine Peel, Chen Pi
Chinese Licorice Root, Gan Cao
Coptis, Huang Lian

This formula clears heat toxin, which is of the result of viral infections.

If you choose to try Chinese herbs, you will find there are several different types. The formula called Long Dan Xie Gan Wan, is the pellet version of Long Dan Xie Gan Tang. The pills are sold over the counter in Chinese grocery stores. The pellets are usually not as strong as capsules and tablets. The only brand of pellets I personally use or prescribe is called Ever Spring.

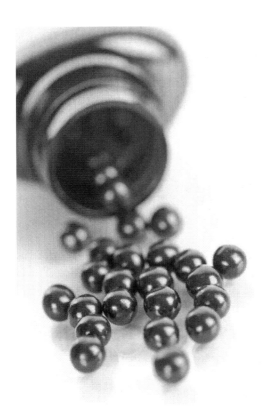

St. John's Wort

St. John's Wort can be used topically as an essential oil to relieve pain, and it can be taken internally. It weakens the protein shell of the virus. This is usually used to treat depression, but it is also effective against all herpes viruses. Please refer to the topical pain reliever chapter.

I know this is a large list of supplements, but I wanted to give you multiple treatment options. Most acupuncturists will have Long Dan Xie Gan Tang in stock. This is a classic herbal formula. There has also been a lot of research confirming its effectiveness against all types of herpes viruses. I would recommend seeking the help of an acupuncturist if you can. If they do not have experience treating this disease, you can refer them to this book.

If you would like *to* study antiviral herbs in more depth, the book *Herbal Antivirals* by Stephen Harrod Buhner is excellent. This book includes information on different types of viruses, and which herb is most recommended to treat that. Although herbs have a much broader spectrum application than pharmaceuticals, each herb has specific actions that will make it a better choice to treat a disease.

Short List Summary

If I were treating myself with things I could buy online, I would buy olive leaf extract and take 2 capsules every 2 hours. I would also take high doses of L-lysine, as this is a well-known treatment for all types of herpes. I would take vitamin C as often as I could. I believe these are the most important supplements in this category.

SHINGLES RELIEF

Chapter 5

Best Natural Pain Relievers

There are many supplements that relieve pain effectively. In my experience, people react differently to everything, so if one supplement does not work for you, you should try another one. I have been prescribing Chinese herbal medicine to treat pain for over 20 years. The results can be amazing.

I am including many natural pain relievers. I am not suggesting you need to take all of them. Each person will be at a different stage of shingles. You might also find that a supplement relieves your pain at one stage, and at a later phase it does not work. That is why it is good to have multiple options.

Immune Health

Your general health will impact the effectiveness of each remedy. You must have enough energy to heal. That is why it takes longer for people over 70 to heal than someone who is 30. For many issues, it will take three times as long to heal if the person is over 70. Even being over 50 will slow healing. Your general health is your ability to get enough sleep, your energy level, and the amount of stress you experience. All of these issues can be treated. Please refer to the "Prevent Future Shingles" chapter for information on how to improve energy levels so you do not get shingles again.

It has become fairly common for people to get shingles more than once. I believe it is because our modern immune systems are not as healthy due to stress, lack of sleep, and the chemicals we are exposed to. Regardless of the cause of pain, there is a way to treat it naturally.

After you get shingles, you will often meet a lot of people who have had it, or know someone who did. Prior to my mom getting shingles, I did not hear a lot about it. I have now heard of people in their twenties getting shingles multiple times. I have also heard of people suffering for years with nerve pain after shingles. Please remember that no matter what stage you are in, there is a way to treat the pain. Whether it is herbs, enzymes, wet cupping, or acupuncture, there is an answer.

Ginger Root

If taken in large enough amounts, Ginger Root can be a very effective pain reliever. You can buy ginger root as a supplement at most stores these days. Most products are raw ginger root that is ground up and encapsulated. That means you have to take more capsules to get the same effect. I prefer to take Planetary Herbal Full Spectrum Ginger. This is ginger extract, which means the ginger root is boiled, and the liquid from that is dried and made into a tablet.

It is hard to say what the exact comparison would be, but you can usually count on a three to one ratio. One ginger extract tablet equals 4 capsules of the raw root, but that varies between brands. It is harder to find ginger extract at stores, so I would not hesitate to buy the raw root from Nature's Way, or Solaray. Jarrow makes a good ginger root extract also.

Ginger root seemed to be one of the best options for shingles pain. I think it is because it also kills viruses. It can be used at the first stage of a cold or flu. It also helps relieve allergy symptoms. Although there are herbal formulas that are stronger, ginger is helpful. For ginger root to be effective on shingles, a higher dosage needs to be taken. Four capsules of the extract at a time is a good start.

Enzymes

A good option to treat pain is systemic enzymes. The reason is that since your body makes its own enzymes, side effects are less likely. Your body makes enzymes to digest your food. It also makes enzymes for cellular repair.

When you are injured, the tissue is damaged. Any type of inflammation or pain will cause scar tissue. The damaged tissue has to be broken down, so the tissue has healthy blood flow. Oxygenated blood is important to tissue health.

Any area of your body that is purple, or red, such as shingles skin, is not getting oxygen. That will

ALWAYS hurt. The goal is to restore healthy blood flow with supplements. If this is not enough, you need some sort of manual therapy to speed healing. Acupuncture, wet cupping, plum blossom therapy, and moxa all increase blood flow to speed healing.

Enzymes dissolve scar tissue. They break down damaged tissue. Your body can only make so much of these. If you eat food that is hard to digest, your body uses most of your enzymes to digest your food. There are not enough enzymes left over to clean up inflamed or damaged tissue. You can easily take supplements with enzymes in them to speed healing and relieve pain.

It is most effective to take enzymes on an empty stomach, so they can be absorbed more quickly. Any enzymes you take on a full stomach will first be used to digest the meal in your stomach. Take enzymes 30 minutes before a meal, or one to two hours after a meal.

Bromelain

Bromelain is an enzyme derived from pineapples. It is a very effective pain reliever. It dissolves damaged tissue in your body. A small dose of bromelain can be very effective. The key is to buy a supplement that has higher active units. The number of milligrams means nothing. The active units per capsule tells you how strong the supplement is. The higher the number, the stronger it is.

I typically recommend at least 2,000 GDU, or active units for bromelain. I like the Source Naturals brand. They make both tablets and capsules. Some people prefer capsules, and some tablets. I prefer tablets.

Doctor's Best brand makes a product with 3,000 GDU per capsule. This is also a good option. I would start with one capsule at a time, and see if that is enough to relieve pain. You do not want to take too much at one time, because it could irritate your stomach lining if it stays in it too long.

Enzymes can be taken long term to treat most types of pain. This is not temporary pain relief. The enzymes go into your bloodstream and break down inflammation and scar tissue, for long term relief. One capsule in the morning might relieve your pain all day.

FYI Restore

This product from the Garden of Life is one of the most effective natural pain relievers. In addition to bromelain, it has other types of enzymes that break down scar tissue. Serrapeptase, and nattokinase make this product much stronger to break down damaged tissue than bromelain taken alone. *Nattokinase* is an enzyme that is very popular in Japan to break down blood clots. It dissolves fibrin in the blood.

A few years ago I injured my leg and FYI Restore was the only product that relieved the pain for me. I normally would use one of the many herbal formulas used in Chinese medicine to treat the pain, but they did not work in this case. I took three to four capsules of FYI Restore at a time, usually twice a day.

Enzymes are measured using different types of units. This makes it harder to compare between brands. The FYI Restore has Bromelain 4,500,000 FCC PU, Protease 35,000 HUT, Nattokinase 500 FU, Serratiopeptidase 10,000 U, and Papain 500,000 FCC PU. You will notice that the Serrapeptase in FYI Restore is measured in a different type of unit than the Doctor's Best brand. That is another reason it is important to use top quality brands.

Quality supplement companies use optimal levels of ingredients. You do not have to worry about the amounts given. If you go to your local discount supercenter to buy your bromelain, they will have a much lower amount of active units per capsule. So it is not as inexpensive as you think. You are not getting as much for your money.

Serrapeptase

This enzyme is made by silkworms to digest their cocoons. It is technically called Serratio Peptidase. It is a natural pain reliever. It can be used in the same way as FYI Restore. You might find that you benefit more with one enzyme formulation than another you have tried. Doctor's Best brand makes a product with 120,000 units per capsule. The FYI Restore product has 10,000 SPU units per capsule.

Enzyme Warning

If you are taking blood thinners, I do not suggest taking supplemental enzymes, unless your health care provider recommends it. This also applies to all herbs. I have yet to find an herb that did not reduce blood viscosity in one way or another which could interact with pharmaceuticals. If you are on any medication, your doctor should be consulted. Enzymes are not likely to cause a problem on their own, but no one knows what they will do when combined with medications.

Enzymes act on non-living tissue only. Although if you take too much, it could irritate your stomach lining, although this is not common.

Myelin Sheath Support

Planetary Herbals also makes a formula that is designed for the myelin sheath. The myelin sheath is the protective coating on the outside of the nerves. When the nerves are damaged, whether by injury or by the shingles virus, the nerves need to be repaired. They need the raw materials, such as the B vitamins, and DHA. You will find information on that in the Post Herpetic Neuralgia chapter.

I do like this formula. The only thing I don't like about it is that it has Asian Ginseng Root Extract. This is also called Chinese or Panax Ginseng. This is not recommended for people who have high blood pressure. There is no way to know if this will increase your blood pressure, as every herb affects people differently. I do not personally recommend testing this product if you have high blood pressure. Ginseng is a great energy tonic, but there are many other herbs that can be used to boost energy that do not have the risk that Asian Ginseng does.

The ingredients are a lot of vitamins and the following herbs: Elderberry fruit, Amla fruit, Asian Ginseng Root Extract, Tienchi Ginseng Root, Hawthorn Berry Extract, Shilajit Mineral Resin Extract, Bromelain, Phellodendron Bark, Guggul Extract, Chebulic Myrobalan Fruit, Boswellia Serrata Gum Resin Extract, Licorice Root Extract, Ashwagandha Root Extract, Turmeric Rhizome Extract, Chinese Salvia Root, Lion's Mane Mycelia, Belleric Myrobalan Fruit, Astragalus Root Extract, Gotu Kola Aerial Parts Extract, Ginger Root, Black Pepper Fruit, Long

Pepper Fruit, Fennel Seed, Asafetida Gum Resin, and Boron Chelate.

 Most of these herbs are natural anti-inflammatory herbs. They improve blood flow also, which speeds healing. This product also has lion's mane, which helps to regenerate the nerves. This is also a brain tonic. There is more about this in the Post Herpetic Neuralgia chapter. Other than the Asian Ginseng, I love this formula for nerve regeneration. I know the ginseng is to boost energy and speed healing, but there are too many people with high blood pressure. I prefer codonopsis, astragalus, or cordyceps for people with high blood pressure.

Willow Aid

This is another pain reliever from Planetary Herbals. It contains willow bark, which is where aspirin was originally derived. It is a natural pain reliever, with fewer likely side effects than aspirin. It also contains Corydalis, Dang Gui, Valerian Root, Boswellin Root Extract, and Guggul Extract. Since it has valerian root, I would not take it in the morning. Valerian root is a sedative, and a nervine. It will help relieve nerve pain, but it might make you drowsy. The other herbs in their formula are strong pain relievers.

Corydalis Minor Pain Relief

This formula is from Planetary Herbals. The reason I mention so many formulas from Planetary Herbals is that these products are formulated by an herbalist. Most companies make single herb supplements. Herbs are often more effective when taken in a combination formula.

Corydalis Minor Pain Relief has Hops, Corydalis, Willow Bark Extract, and Ginger Root Extract. Willow Bark, as mentioned before, is the source of aspirin, before it was synthesized chemically. Hops is a natural anti-inflammatory. Hops is a sedative, it can be used for insomnia and anxiety. I would take this in the evening first, to see how the formula affects you.

Inflama-Care

This is my favorite pain reliever from Planetary Herbals. It is very similar to an herbal formula I use as an acupuncturist. The theory behind it is that any type of pain is caused by bad circulation.

When you restore blood flow, the body can heal the affected area.

As long as the area is purple, that shows there is a lack of oxygen in the tissue, so it will continue to hurt as long as it is purple, in most cases. Even if the skin looks healed, if there is still pain, there is a blockage under the surface.

Inflama-Care can resolve the blockage. The herbs dissolve the stagnant blood that does not have enough oxygen. You might have heard of Curcumin. Curcumin is also called Turmeric. Curcumin is the component of the spice Turmeric. This is used to relieve pain. Taking it alone is not as effective as taking it in a formula. This product contains: Turmeric extract, Boswellin, Ginger root, Bromelain, Willow Bark Extract, Chinese Skullcap root extract, Hops Flower Extract, Corydalis, Holy Basil Leaf Extract, Quercetin, Rosemary Leaf Extract, trans-Resveratrols (from Polygonum cuspidatum root extract), Masson Pine Bark Extract, Grape Seed Extract, EGCG from green tea, Lecithin, Black Pepper Fruit Extract (BioPerine).

This formula can be used to treat many types of pain. It contains different types of pain relievers that each address pain. It also contains bromelain, which is a pain relieving enzyme. It is a natural anti-inflammatory.

Chapter 6

Cupping Therapy

Wet cupping was the most effective treatment for my mom's shingles pain. I believe that post herpetic neuralgia is often caused by a residual virus that is affecting the nerve. The virus is not gone yet. It needs to be purged. The day after I wet cupped her, she had a 40% reduction in pain. It continued to improve. More than one treatment was necessary. If caught early, the problem can often be resolved with fewer treatments.

Meaning of Purple Lesions

Shingles lesions are purple. This is one thing that stood out to me as an acupuncturist. Purple always means there is stuck blood in the area. As long as the area is purple, even if it is not visible on the surface, the body cannot resolve the damaged tissue.

Modern medicine does not have a definitive answer about the exact mechanism of nerve damage. The most common theories are:

1. The virus damages the nerves, which causes pain.
2. The virus causes an immune response in the body, which causes the inflammatory response that causes pain.

My personal theory is that although the nerves might be damaged, the pain can be either from tight muscles near the spine, from the nerve irritations, or the virus is still active. The fact that people can recover quickly if given the right treatment, makes me believe that the virus causes an inflammation, which causes pain. If you can help the body to overcome the virus, you can relieve the pain. Once the treatments are done, your body is able to make the virus go dormant again.

In Chinese medicine theory, if tissue is purple, that means there is stagnant blood. That means there is no oxygen in it. Improving blood flow to improve oxygen levels will help your body to function normally again. As long as the lesions are purple, they will hurt, because the body cannot get enough oxygen in the tissue to heal it. The immune complexes in the blood also have to get access to the virus.

It might be that the body is actually protecting you from the active virus by cutting off blood flow to the area. The virus damages the nerves, so either the nerves cause the damage that makes the skin purple, or the body is protecting you from the virus. I suggest taking anti-viral herbs until the virus is completely gone and there is no pain, or any other symptom.

Even if the area is not purple, you can still use wet cupping to treat it. Just treat the most painful area. It does not hurt as much as you think, and it will resolve the shingles so the pain will finally end.

How Cupping Works
Cupping is a technique used in Chinese medicine to treat many ailments. One of the most common

things it is used for is to treat pain. You might have seen pictures of famous people with purple marks on their bodies. These marks are often in a circular shape.

The objective of cupping is to increase circulation. The ancient style of cupping is called Fire Cupping. A piece of cotton is soaked in alcohol, and is set on fire. The cotton is put inside the glass cup for a second. This creates a vacuum. The cup itself does not get hot. It is applied to the area to be treated. When the cup is left on the skin, the suction pulls the skin up and the stagnant blood is pulled to the surface. This enables your body to resolve the stagnant blood. If there is no stagnant blood, you will usually not see any purple marks, unless you leave the cups on too long.

Cupping with Plastic Cups and a Vacuum Pump

A modern way to do cupping is with plastic cups, and a pump. The cups have a rubber valve on them where the vacuum pump is attached. The pump pulls air out of the cup, while the cup is on the area to be treated.

Silicone Cups

A newer way to cup is silicone cups. There is no suction device required. All you do is squeeze the cup tightly and place on the skin. That provides all the suction you need. If you get enough suction, the skin underneath the cup turns purple. The areas that were lanced will have a drop of blood sitting on the surface.

Wet Cupping

This is the technique that is very effective for shingles. I did not know about this until two months after my mom got the shingles. I wish I had known in the beginning. I believe I could have resolved her shingles within a few days. This technique is not very well known.

Although this will seem strange to you, and I agree it is a bit tough, it will relieve the pain and resolve the virus quickly. I learned about this technique being effective for shingles in an acupuncture group I belong to on Facebook. There were many different techniques that people used successfully, including moxa, plum blossom therapy, and acupuncture. Your acupuncturist might get great results with another method. I did not. The age and general health of a patient affects the effectiveness of different treatments.

You might be familiar with the concept of bloodletting. The Chinese method of bloodletting is not the same as the one where large amounts of blood are removed from the patient. Small drops are all you need. This technique is not as widespread as it should be. Since many acupuncturists have not been exposed to this technique, I will explain it in detail.

Piercing the Skin

Your acupuncturist can pierce the skin with a safety lancet. There are several ways to pierce the skin. Some acupuncturists use different types of needles. The lancets that diabetics use to draw blood to test their blood sugar are not sharp enough. They are used on the fingertips, where it is easy to draw blood.

The size that works best for this technique is 17 gauge. There are safety lancets that are a one-time use only. You can buy them in boxes of 100. The type I bought was McKesson "Push-Button Safety Lancets, 17G Blade." I like using the safety lancets, because I am new to this technique and I feel more comfortable with this. Acupuncturists who have been trained in this technique will have their own preferred way of piercing the skin. Some use hypodermic needles, and others three edge needles.

Safety Lancets

The safety lancet has a plastic safety tip that needs to be removed. Place the lancet on the skin and press down firmly. The lancet pops out once, pierces the skin, and then pops back inside. So it is very safe. There is only a tiny amount of blood until you apply the cups with suction. I only left the cups on for a few minutes. After the cup was removed, I placed a tissue on the area to soak up the blood.

Wet Cupping Mom

The first time I did wet cupping on my mom's shingles, I was not as aggressive, and my mom did not have much benefit. This was the last treatment option for us after two months of herbs, and other acupuncture techniques. She was not able to stand plum blossom therapy, and other techniques were not fast enough, so I tried again. She is 79 years old, and I believe that was why the other therapies we tried did not work for her. She was depleted after having the flu a few weeks prior. The second time I was more aggressive, because I had nothing to lose.

The next day she was almost pain free. The shock pains were gone. The lesions started to shrink. I waited two days to treat her again. I had her take high quantities of Cordyceps Power, and Cordyceps tea to build her energy up to fight the virus.

Gloves should be worn when doing this technique. The blood that comes out will have active shingles virus in it, so it is hazardous waste. The cups should also be either thrown away, or sterilized with Sporox II. The best option for this is to buy plastic cupping sets with 24 cups in them. This will enable you to cover all the lesions.

Wet cupping can be used as soon as the patient realizes she has shingles. It is not necessary to wait for the lesions to scab over, which usually takes two to three weeks. I wish I had used this technique at the beginning of my mom's shingles. It would have saved her a lot of pain. This technique is not commonly known in America. I called a Chinese acupuncturist I know for advice and he suggested moxibustion.

I belong to several online groups for acupuncturists, where we share treatment advice, and give each other advice on tough cases. This book includes information from these groups, as well as multiple books and online resources. Moxibustion, far infrared heat lamp, plum blossom therapy, and herbal remedies were discussed as treatment options. The treatments in this book are effective for many acupuncturists.

Sarah K. Roell, LAc, is a licensed acupuncturist in Columbus, Ohio. She learned this technique in China. She said that shingles was one of her favorite things to treat, because she got great results with it. She can be reached at Dynamic Flow Acupuncture. Her detailed technique is below.

Sarah uses a hypodermic needle to pierce the skin, she feels that is less painful than a safety lancet. The hypodermic needle will enable deeper piercing, and more precise location. The following information is paraphrased:

1. Bleed the largest, most angry looking vesicles in the area, and apply a cup immediately. She usually bleeds 5-8 vesicles under each cup.

2. Continue treating areas to cover the entire rash, adding as many cups as the patient's constitution will allow. The number of cups will vary with the size of the rash. You can place the cups directly next to each other all along the rash.

3. Keep the cups on until the blood stops flowing, usually 10 or so minutes. She says that she does not have an exact timeframe on how long to leave the cups on. She leaves the cups on as long as the blood is moving, which is usually about 10 minutes.

4. Remove the cups and wipe the areas with witch hazel.

5. If you were not able to bleed all the main vesicles, do another round of bleeding and cupping to cover the areas that were blocked by the cups on the first round.

The pain level should be decreased after treatment, and the pain should continue to improve over the next day or so. Generally, the pain will drop to low to none within 24 hours after treatment.

If the symptoms are not gone, additional bleeding and cupping should be done. Choose different areas where the pain is located.

If you treat someone who has residual nerve pain, but no visible rash, treat the areas that are most painful. If there is no visible rash, it will take more treatments to achieve full results, as it will be harder to locate the affected areas.

The age of the patient does not seem to matter in how fast the therapy works. The length of time they have been dealing with shingles can affect the number of treatments necessary for complete relief. The best results are when treatment is done on active pustules. If they have already cleared, you will not be able to get all the spots you need to treat. (This would just mean you need more treatments to get it all, rather than complete relief in one or two treatments.)

The normally recommended time to leave the cups on is 10-15 minutes. The goal of this therapy is not to extract the maximum amount of blood. I got the best results after leaving the cups on for 15 minutes. I believe it is the fact that the cup pulls blood flow into the area, which stimulates the body to heal it.

Some acupuncturists use plum blossom therapy for shingles and it is very effective. I believe that a fast resolution is necessary for this pain, so I prefer the more aggressive approach. In my opinion, plum blossom therapy is more painful than wet cupping. Please refer to the plum blossom chapter for information on this technique.

This information is not widely known in America. I found one video showing a patient who had plum blossom therapy, combined wet cupping, rather than using a lancet or other piercing needle. I posted this on my website, at www.acupunctureexplained.com.

I know that wet cupping will sound rather gruesome to most people. Shingles pain is more painful than childbirth, according to people who have had it. I was just desperate enough to try this technique, and it worked for us. If you have not had a complete resolution of your pain with other methods, you might consider getting wet cupping as an option.

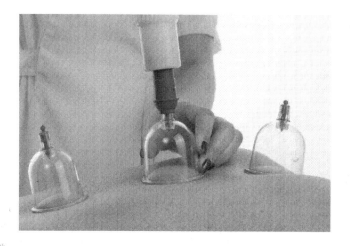

SHINGLES RELIEF

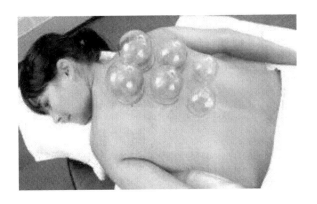

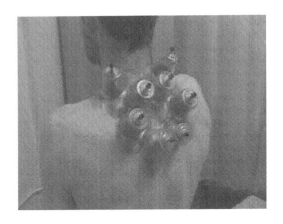

Chapter 7

Heat Vs Ice Therapy – What Works

The shingles rash feels hot. Some might recommend you apply ice to relieve the pain. That is not recommended in Chinese medicine theory. It has also been proven to be ineffective. The reason is that applying ice will chill the area and reduce blood flow. This slows down the rate of swelling, but your body will fight against this. The swelling is caused by your body sending inflammatory chemicals into the area so it can heal itself. There is modern research supporting the theory that ice therapy, as most people use it, is not as effective as many people think.

Heat therapy relieves pain. Heat improves blood flow, and relaxes muscles. Unless you specifically search online for the words "heat" and "shingles," you will not find anything recommending applying heat. I found various posts from people who had shingles who felt a lot better when they took warm showers, or applied moist heat. Be very careful to not overheat the area. Use very gentle warmth, not heat.

Far Infrared or TDP Lamp Therapy

One therapy that is commonly used by acupuncturists is called far infrared heat. The heat lamp is called either a frar infrared lamp, or a TDP lamp. This is using a special heat lamp that has a mineral plate on it. It penetrates deeper into the skin than other types of heat. It is helpful for any type of pain. That alone can be enough to treat and resolve pain. It is very important not to overdo it. Be gentle on yourself when using heat therapy. TDP lamp therapy improves blood flow, and relieves pain. If your immune system is strong enough, it might help to resolve the virus.

Chapter 8

Plum Blossom Therapy

Plum blossom therapy is an ancient Chinese healing technique. The device you use is similar to a hammer. There are seven prongs on the end of the hammer. This device is also called a Seven Star Needle. You simply tap firmly on the affected shingles.

This is one of the most commonly used and effective ways to treat shingles. It is not painless. However, you could technically treat yourself. An acupuncturist friend of mine started getting shingles on her knee. She used her plum blossom hammer and hit all over her shingles lesion. It went away and never became full-blown shingles. You have to be fairly aggressive with this. The goal is to pierce the skin enough to stimulate blood flow to the surface.

I consulted with many acupuncturists on Facebook, and many people use this, and one person said he knows a medical doctor who uses it. It is surprising that it is so effective, but it is one more way that Chinese medicine is shown to have the answer to just about any health problem.

Each hammer costs about a dollar. I would not re-use the hammer. Use a fresh one every time the treatment is done. Treat daily. I would combine this with anti-viral herbs.

Seven star needle, or plum blossom therapy pierces the skin, which improves blood flow. I believe that piercing the skin with the hammer makes it easier for your immune system to attack the virus. Some viruses are able to hide themselves from the immune system.

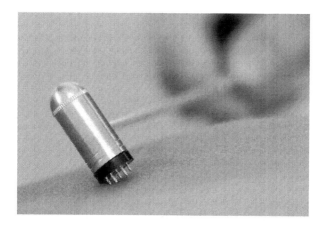

The hammer in this image is metal. Most hammers are plastic. When this therapy is done, viral particles will be released. Please take precautions.

According to a book about the Chinese medicine treatment of shingles, *Acupuncture and Moxibustion for Herpes Zoster*, by Zhao Ji-ping, and Wang Jun, this therapy is useful for both acute herpes zoster, and post-herpetic neuralgia. It says to treat the affected areas, including the spine points. It is seen as purging toxins in Chinese medicine theory.

If the red or purple shingles lesions are already resolved, you can tap where the lesions were located. That is why it is easier to treat the virus when it first attacks. Do not give up. Even without obvious lesions, you can get results. It will just take longer.

This therapy is pretty simple. This is one of the most commonly used therapies to treat shingles.

Chapter 9

Moxibustion Therapy

Moxibustion is an ancient Chinese medicine treatment. It is commonly used to treat pain, although it can also be used to stimulate acupuncture points. The most common usage is for back pain. It is helpful to restore circulation in the back, which relieves pain. If you do research on this, you will often find images of people with things on their back that have smoke coming out of them. That is moxa.

Moxa is the name of the herb that is burned. It is also called mugwort, or Artemisia. It is also called wormwood leaf.

The herb is rolled into the shape of a cigar, and lit. The moxa heat rapidly relieves coldness that settles in areas of pain. I used moxibustion on my dad after his stroke 20 years ago. After the stroke, his left leg was cold to the touch, and he was limping. I knew that if his leg was cold, that there would be a reduction in blood flow in the area. Unless I could restore the normal temperature in his leg, he would not be able to walk normally.

The only tools I had with me at the time were moxa and needles. I did moxa on the back of his leg for a couple of hours, and he was able to walk almost normally after that. I was able to treat him the week after his stroke. I quickly restored healthy circulation with the moxa and needles.

If you know someone who had a stroke, I would suggest they try acupuncture. The sooner you get treatment, the better your results are. There are many types of acupuncture that are used to restore normal function after a stroke. Scalp acupuncture, and abdominal acupuncture are also popular for this.

Moxibustion works on shingles also. I have read of numerous accounts of people using this to treat shingles. Moxa each area for 15 minutes. Do not overheat. I also do not recommend moxa spray for this. It has other herbs in it that are not appropriate for shingles.

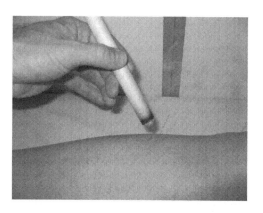

There are different types of moxa. There is pure moxa, which is just Artemisia, and moxa combined with other herbs. It can be combined with herbs that tonify the kidneys. There is also smokeless moxa, which is carbonized mugwort herb. That is what I used on my dad. It is like a piece of charcoal in a cigar shape. You have to light it with a candle, because it takes about 5-10 minutes to be fully lit. Once it is lit, it glows like lit charcoal. You have to tap every minute or so to get the ashes off the moxa, so they do not fall on the patient.

Moxibustion treatment can easily cause insomnia. The herb is very strong. A lot of acupuncturists become allergic to it, because they use it so much. I don't know very many acupuncturists who use moxa. In addition, pure moxa smells like marijuana when it is burned. The smokeless type does not smell like that though. Some people think their local acupuncturist is smoking marijuana in another room when they use moxa.

If you find an acupuncturist who has experience with treating shingles with moxa, that can be a good treatment option. There are many ways to treat a disease, and I do not discount one type over another. I did not get good results with this therapy for shingles. However, I wanted to mention it so you would be familiar with it if you ran across it. I know very good acupuncturists who use this method successfully.

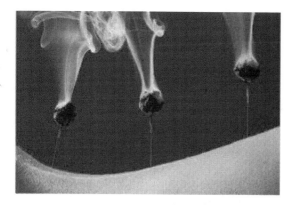

This image shows moxa on the tip of the needle. The moxa warms the needle.

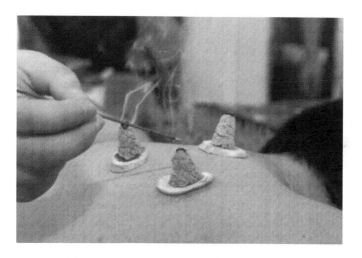

This image shows ginger moxa. Slices of ginger are placed on the area to be treated, and moxa is placed on top and lit. There are many ways that moxa can be used to treat disease.

Chapter 10

Post Herpetic Neuralgia - Healing Damaged Nerves

Post herpetic neuralgia (PHN) is the residual nerve pain that occurs in about 20% of people who suffer from shingles. This is the nerve pain that lingers after the skin lesions have been resolved. It can last for months, or even years.

Symptoms of PHN include:
- Sharp burning, shooting, or stabbing pain
- Sensitivity to touch, often it hurts to wear clothes that touch the body
- Burning, throbbing, or aching pains
- Sensitivity to changes in temperature
- Itching
- Headaches

- Possible muscle weakness
- Falling easily
- Numbness or tingling
- Loss of balance or coordination

Some pain that is classified as post herpetic neuralgia is caused by tight muscles. I met a woman who had suffered for years with residual pain. Four acupuncture treatments were all she needed to be pain free. It is not possible to know if the pain is caused by tight muscles only. If tight muscles are pressing on the nerves, the acupuncture will easily relieve that pain. I also believe that doing acupuncture on the affected area will improve blood flow and immune complexes into the area, so your body can deal with the virus.

Is Post Herpetic Neuralgia Caused by the Residual Herpes Virus?

In the antiviral chapter, I mentioned that I believe that a lot of the post herpetic neuralgia is actually caused by a residual virus. The virus is still active. So in addition to taking supplements that heal the nerves, I would make sure that the virus has been treated by herbs like Olive Leaf Extract, and others mentioned in that chapter.

There is an article on www.sciencedaily.com called "Antiviral Drugs May Help Relieve Nerve Pain Related to Shingles." This report originated in JAMA, or the Journal of the American Medical Association. The article states that "Post herpetic neuralgia can last for months or years, and affects as many as one million people in the United States." This article concludes that anti-viral drugs can be used to relieve post herpetic neuralgia, which confirms the theory that a lot of this pain is caused by an active viral infection.

A study was done by Dianna Quan, MD, at the University of Colorado and Health Sciences Center, Denver. They administered antiviral therapy to 15 patients. They received 10 milligrams of an antiviral medication intravenously every eight hours for 14 days. They also took three 1,000 milligram pills of valacyclovir, an anti-viral drug, per day for one month. After one month of therapy, 53 percent of the patients reported that their pain had reduced significantly.

In my experience, herbal antivirals are very effective. With the correct formula, viruses can be resolved very effectively. The best thing about herbs and vitamins is that there is usually no downside.

Treat the Cause of Pain

In order to resolve a health problem, you need to know what is causing it. There are many supplements that treat the viral aspect of shingles, but there are also many supplements that can improve the healing of damaged nerves. Some herbs heal the nerves, and treat the virus at the same time.

My first choice to treat shingles is to do either plum blossom therapy, or wet cupping. In most cases this will resolve the outbreak much faster than depending on supplements. However, the virus damages the nerves. It is also helpful to take supplements to speed healing.

DHA

DHA is a type of fat that is derived from krill oil, or fish oil. The myelin sheath is the fatty insulation that protects your nerves. It is 75% fat. If you want to repair the nerves, you need a good quality oil. DHA is also good for your brain. It is a great memory booster. The other 25% of the nerve tissue is protein. The vitamin C you take will help you to produce the collagen necessary to heal that.

Acetyl L-Carnitine, also called ALC

This type of L-Carnitine is one of the most important supplements mentioned to treat post herpetic neuralgia, along with DHA. L-Carnitine balances your blood sugar, helps you burn fat, and the acetyl type of Carnitine reduces nerve pain. Studies on this supplement show that it relieves numbness and pain, and helps to repair damaged nerves. This supplement is often cited in research on treating diabetic neuropathy. ALC also improves brain function, and memory.

Alpha Lipoic Acid, also called ALA

Lipoic acid is an antioxidant used to treat diabetic neuropathy. It is both fat and water soluble, which means it can penetrate cell membranes

Buying Effective Medicinal Mushrooms

Medicinal mushrooms are very effective to improve nerve health. They are also deep immune tonics, as well as having many other health benefits. It is important to know what part of the mushroom was used to make the supplement. Mushroom supplements are often made with the mycelium part of the mushroom. The mycelium is the new growth, or the roots of the mushroom. This is often not the strongest part to use medicinally. Some products combine the mycelium and the fruiting body, so you get the benefits of both. If they do not state on the label that the fruiting body was used, you can assume they used the mycelium, because it is a lot less expensive than the fruiting body.

The fruiting body is the mature mushroom. Mushroom mycelium supplements are often very high in rice powder content. The mushroom is grown on rice, and the immature part, or mycelium, is more rice than mushroom. You will notice it is very pale and bland smelling. The fruiting body is much stronger smelling, and darker.

Always be sure to by a mushroom *extract*. Taking raw mushroom will not be very effective. The mushrooms need to be broken down to be effective. The most common way to do this is to boil them.

There are several good brands of mushroom fruiting body available right now. Some brands include Freshcap, Wild Shroom, and Real Mushrooms.

Lion's Mane Mushroom

This mushroom is a deep immune tonic. It helps to rebuild the immune system that has been depleted by an active virus. Your body uses a lot of resources to protect you from viruses. After the outbreak is over, the immune system will need to be rebuilt. The more you can focus on restoring your health with supplements, the less likely you are to get the virus again. Lion's mane also improves brain function, and helps to repair nerve tissue. This supplement is currently being studied to determine how it can help cognitive function. The mushroom actually looks like a brain.

Reishi Mushroom

Reishi mushroom is a deep immune tonic. It is also a nervine, which means it can calm the nerves down. Some sources say it affects the herpes virus directly. I like the Reishi Mushroom Supreme product from Planetary Formulas. Reishi mushroom is one of the most frequently mentioned mushrooms to treat and prevent shingles.

Nerve Damage

Herpes zoster damages the nerves. Although I believe that residual nerve pain can be a result of an active virus, there are many supplements that will help the nerves heal faster. There are herbs that are considered to be "nervines". These herbs calm the nerves down. They can also be used to treat anxiety and insomnia. The intense pain of shingles is very stressful to the body. The body is in shock.

Taking vitamins, minerals, and essential fatty acids will give your body the building blocks it needs to repair damaged tissue. Nerves are about 75% fat. The myelin sheath, which coats the nerves and acts as an insulator, can be repaired. The following supplements are used to repair the body.

A Note about Vitamin Brands

It is not a good idea to take cheap vitamins from a big box store. These vitamins are not absorbed well. I have had a lot of experience over the years of patients using inexpensive products that do not work. Once the quality product is used, it is easy to tell the difference. An example of this is grape seed extract.

Nature's Way OPC brand is the type that uses the same component of the grape seed extract that has been proven to treat varicose veins, and other weak collagen in the body. Jacques Masquelier is the person who did the original research on this. When patients bleed after acupuncture, I know they need grape seed extract, because their veins are weak.

I receive no compensation whatsoever from the brands I recommend. I have used many supplements over the years, and I do a lot of research on which brands are the best.

B Vitamins
The B vitamins are very important to heal the nerves. They are also rapidly depleted when you are under stress. Adrenal fatigue is caused by

intense stress. This will increase the time it takes to recover. B Vitamins and vitamin C are the most important for your adrenals and nerves. My favorite B vitamins are from the Garden of Life. They are called *Raw B*. Each vitamin is fermented and enzyme processed to ensure you absorb it well. I have tested many brands of vitamins over the years, and I can actually feel a difference pretty quickly when I take the Raw series of vitamins.

The B vitamins can be very effective on their own. I met a woman who recovered from post herpetic neuralgia using B vitamins alone. They acted as pain relievers for her.

Benfotiamine (Vitamin B-1)

This type of B vitamins is fat soluble. Most B vitamins are water soluble, which might affect how they are absorbed into the cells. This type of B-1 is prescribed in Germany to treat sciatica and other types of nerve pain. I don't know if this special type of B-1 is completely necessary, or if the regular B vitamin formula is enough. I wanted to mention it, and you can decide for yourself. I think it might be worthwhile to use it for a while.

Vitamin B 12

This is the number one vitamin to boost energy levels. Doctors used to give people B 12 shots when they were suffering from fatigue. Unfortunately, that is not common these days, but you can take vitamin pills. It is important to take the best type of B 12. There are two types. There is cyanocobalamin, and methylcobalamin. The methylcobalamin type is absorbed better than the cyanocobalamin type.

I take the Garden of Life Raw B 12. It is fairly expensive, but I can feel the difference, so I think it is well absorbed. If you can get a B-12 shot from your doctor, that would be a nice option. Many people are B 12 deficient, and they will feel better energy levels when they take this. I would combine it with a B vitamin complex formula to ensure balance.

My research indicates that B 12 restores healthy blood flow to the nerves, and improves the production of myelin. Myelin is the fatty coating on your nerves. It is like wire insulation. If it is damaged, the nerves do not function normally.

Alpha Lipoic Acid

Diabetics are advised to use alpha lipoic acid to treat and prevent nerve pain. By the way, acupuncture treats diabetic neuropathy very well. In my opinion, no one should have a limb amputated before trying a course of acupuncture. Acupuncture restores healthy blood flow to treat nerve pain. Once circulation is restored, pain goes away.

Gotu Kola

Gotu Kola is an Indian herb. It does not contain caffeine. It is also called Centella, the Latin name is Centella Asiatica. People often think it is kola nut, which does have caffeine. Gotu Kola is a nervine. It is one of the most effective herbs to treat anxiety and stress. It also improves memory. It is used to treat varicose veins, because it improves the repair of damaged collagen. I like the Nature's Way brand, and the Solaray brand. Three capsules is a good dosage, since this is not an extract, it is the raw herb.

Solaray – Nerve Blend Sp-14

There is an herbal blend that combines several herbal nervines in one product. If you try to buy a bottle of each type of herb that relieves nerve pain, you will not be able to take them all. Herbs are also often more effective when combined. This formula is made by Solaray, which is my favorite herb company. They always have great quality, and they process the herbs properly, which means they work better.

Nerve Blend combines valerian root, passion flower, wood betony, ginger root, hops, skullcap, chamomile, and blessed thistle. You might recognize valerian root as a sleep herb. It helps you sleep by relaxing your muscles. Chamomile is a popular tea to relieve stress also. All these herbs help relax the nerves. Ginger root is a natural anti-inflammatory, and a great pain reliever. Ginger is often used in formulas to harmonize the other herbs. It also improves digestion.

Ginger can be taken as a natural pain reliever on its own. It is one of the best herbs to keep in your medicine cabinet. The dosage of this is 2 capsules. I would start with that, then consider 3-4 if 2 is not enough. It will help you recover from the effects of shingles pain. It will take a little time to calm your nervous system down.

Due to the high amount of valerian root in this product, please be aware it might make you drowsy. I do not think this formula is a magic bullet for nerve pain, but it might relieve enough pain for some people to make it worthwhile.

Calcium and Magnesium

Magnesium deficiency is very common. Over 80% of us do not get enough magnesium. Your body needs magnesium to relax your muscles. If you do not get enough of it, your body cannot relax. In order to absorb calcium, you must have magnesium and other cofactors. You cannot absorb the calcium in dairy products, because it is not bio-available. It is bound to the protein and not well absorbed.

An uncle of mine has Type 1 Diabetes. He had nerve pain so bad that he could not ride in a car. This is diabetic neuropathy. He took a calcium supplement and relieved most of his nerve pain. It was a miracle supplement for him. If you do not have all the vitamins and minerals your body needs to function normally, you cannot be completely healthy.

One of the most common causes of calcium and magnesium deficiencies is soda pop. If you drink soft drinks, read the label. Most of them contain phosphoric acid in them. That gives the product a tart taste, and it also enables you to drink massive quantities of liquid sugar. It also is an acid, and it must be buffered to prevent it from doing damage to your body. Your body uses minerals to buffer this acid. If you do not have enough calcium in your blood, it will pull calcium from your bones. I believe that is one reason that osteoporosis is becoming common.

Even one soft drink a day, whether it is diet or regular soda, can be enough to cause bone pain. You can feel this ache in joints that have been injured. For example, if you broke a toe at some point, or had an issue with your teeth, you can feel an ache when your body pulls calcium from the areas where bone was recently deposited. I know acupuncturists who strongly suggest magnesium supplements for all their patients who have pain. I have also had patients with chronic pain have a 50% reduction in their pain levels after taking a good supplement.

Raw Calcium Supplement

My favorite calcium and magnesium supplement is Raw Calcium from Garden of life. This will supply calcium, magnesium, vitamin D, and other cofactors your body needs to make bone. This is a marine derived mineral formula that has been shown to help people with osteoporosis or osteopenia, which is the stage where you are on your way to osteoporosis. The dosage is four pills a day. If you have drunk soft drinks regularly, you might consider a higher dosage. If you have bone pain, it might be relieved quickly with this product.

Calcium is also necessary for nerve function. If you are low in calcium, your nerves cannot function properly. Research has been done on the effect that calcium has on nerve healing, and nerve function. Your body can become acidic if you do not have enough calcium. This can cause chronic pain that is not relieved with medications. If you have chronic pain of any sort, consider taking multi-vitamins from the Garden of Life Raw line. You do not know which vitamin might be causing your chronic pain.

Calcium cannot be absorbed without magnesium and other cofactors such as vitamin D. It is not good to take calcium supplements on their own. They cannot be absorbed, and can cause other health issues.

Vitamin C

The importance of vitamin C cannot be overstated. If your body has enough vitamin C, it will be more able to overcome any virus. I have read numerous articles, even one by Dr. Whitaker, that state that vitamin C is helpful for shingles pain. Some people experience a complete resolution of nerve pain when enough vitamin C is taken.

I also like the lipospheric type of vitamin C. It is more expensive than tablets, but you do not need to take as much, and it is absorbed into the cells faster. I also like Reacta-C from KAL. It is Strontium Calcium Ascorbate. It also has high levels of bioflavonoids, which your body uses to make collagen. They are believed to increase the effectiveness of vitamin C. Even though I have favorite vitamin C supplements, you can take any type of vitamin C.

If you are interested in further research on vitamin C, there are many articles on the website www.peakenergy.com. These articles are written by Dr. Thomas E. Levy, who is an expert on the uses of vitamin C. I believe that the spontaneous recoverys some people get with high doses of vitamin C are a result of activating the immune system, so it can resolve the virus completely. If you don't like taking a lot of pills, Emergen-C makes a good powdered vitamin C.

According to an article on www.betternutrition.com, vitamin C relieves fatigue. According to researchers at the National Institutes of Health, fatigue was one of the first signs of vitamin C depletion. In one study, 44 workers received 6 grams of vitamin C daily. After two weeks their fatigue had decreased by almost one-third. Your body needs enough vitamin C to make important neurotransmitters that regulate mood. According to a recent study in Montreal, almost two thirds of patients in an acute medical ward had low or deficient levels of vitamin C. Taking 1,000 mg of vitamin C daily helped to reduce anger, anxiety, and depression.

Is Post Herpetic Neuralgia Caused by the Active Shingles Virus?

You have to ask yourself why some people get over shingles completely in a few weeks, and other people have pain for months and years. Unless you consider that the virus is still active, it does not make sense. Yes, the nerves are damaged and need to be repaired. You need the appropriate vitamins and fatty acids to repair the nerves, so that can be a factor in the ability to resolve the pain. You also need enough vitality to recover from any illness. Please see the chapter on preventing future shingles attacks.

The lesions can be purple or red for months. What is that? I think it is the active shingles virus that has not been resolved yet. My suspicions were confirmed when I looked for shingles information in a textbook called *The Treatment of Pain with Chinese Herbs and Acupuncture*, which was edited by Sun Peilin. This is a great addition to anyone's library on Chinese Medicine.

In the chapter on axillary pain, one of the diagnoses is "invasion of toxic heat to the channels." Toxic heat is the Chinese way of explaining shingles, in this case. Heat is usually inflammation, but toxic heat is extreme heat. This is often associated with viral invasions. The symptoms and signs of this per this pain book are: Pain with redness, swelling, tenderness and warmth, accompanied by chills, fever, headache, and thirst.

The interesting thing was that an herbal prescription was given, and it was stated that the herbal formula would "reduce the "Fire" and remove toxic heat. When the toxic heat is cleared, and there is no disturbance to the Qi and blood circulation, the pain disappears." That means that when the virus is gone, the pain will go away too. The virus does not actually leave, it goes dormant again.

This section of the book confirms my suspicion that nerve pain caused by shingles is often the result of the virus not being resolved. The virus is not gone. The virus was already smoldering in your body, waiting for your immune system to go down for some reason, so it can reactivate itself. Anti-viral supplements and treatments such as wet cupping, and plum blossom therapy can be used to resolve the viral attack.

There are many Chinese herbal formulas that are used to treat different types of viruses in Chinese medicine. This book recommends a formula called "Wu Wei Xiao Du Yin." This formula is comprised of: Jin Yin Hua, Ye Ju Hua, Pu Gong Ying, Zi Hua Di Ding, and Zi Bei Tian Kui. The translations of these herbs are: Flos Lonicerae, Flos Chysanthemi, Herba Taraxaci (dandelion root), Herba Viola, and Herba Begonia Fibristipulatae. This formula is an anti viral that specifically treats the toxic heat that occurs with shingles.

At this time, modern medicine has not been able to specify exactly the pain of shingles. An article called "Hypotheses on the Pathogenesis of Herpes Zoster-associated Pain," by Gary J. Bennet, PhD, can be found at www.onlinelibrary.wiley.com. Dr. Bennett basically states that there is little direct evidence of what causes the nerve pain of shingles. It could be caused by the damage to the nerves, but it might also be the inflammation caused by the virus.

The lesions of shingles are purple in the beginning of the attack. Your body causes inflammation to heal damaged tissue, which causes the tissue to turn red, or in this case, purple. In Chinese medicine, purple means that there is no blood flow. There is no oxygen in the tissue. Any tissue that is purple is going to hurt.

Chinese Herbs for Viruses

As a side note, there are many herbal formulas that treat viruses, there are hundreds if not thousands to choose from. The formula that most precisely suits the specific viral symptoms and stage of the disease is chosen. A very effective treatment for the common cold or flu is the formula called *Zhong Gan Ling*. I have had success within 24 hours with this formula. It is a modern herbal formula. It is best to treat viral invasions as fast as you can after you contract them, before the virus has a chance to multiply. It basically takes over your body and reproduces itself. The longer you have had it, the more likely you are to develop other problems like bronchitis and pneumonia.

Chapter Summary

It is difficult to take all the supplements that can help PHN. The supplements I would personally focus on are acetyl l-carnitine, Raw Calcium, the

Solaray Nerve Blend herbs, Vitamin C, and Raw B vitamins. Those are the most important.

Pharmaceutical Side Effects

Neurontin (gabapentin) is an anti-epileptic drug that is used to treat seizures. It is also commonly prescribed for the nerve pain from shingles. Some people find it effective, and others do not. My chief concern is how many people take this drug who are unaware of the potential side effects. In my experience, people have side effects from taking drugs and they do not know that is the cause of their symptoms.

According to www.rxlist.com, common side effects of this drug are: dizziness, drowsiness, unsteadiness, memory loss, lack of coordination, difficulty speaking, viral infections, tremors, double vision, fever, unusual eye movements, and jerky movements. This list of side effects is not all inclusive. These are just the most common ones. If you have any symptoms that are unusual for you, please consult your medical doctor. You can also report side effects to the FDA at 1-800-FDA-1088.

SHINGLES RELIEF

Chapter 11

Prevent Future Shingles Attacks, and Recover Your Health

Shingles outbreaks are caused by a weak immune system. Normally your body keeps the virus under control. The herpes virus stays in your body after you get chickenpox. When your immune system is too weak to keep it under control, it is able to attack you again. The key to preventing shingles is to strengthen your immune system, and to boost your energy levels. The supplements in this chapter will also speed healing from current attacks.

If you are a caregiver treating someone with shingles, it would help you a lot to take some immune tonic herbs during the outbreak to reduce the chance of having your own shingles outbreak.

According to the *Mayo Clinic Proceedings* report, the likelihood of getting shingles more than once is most affected by how bad the pain is in the first episode of the disease. If your pain lasts more than 30 days after the initial onset of shingles, you are more likely to get it again. This information is secondary from www.sciencedaily.com.

Most people do not take supplements to improve their immune health, which makes it more likely to get the shingles several times. I believe that if the right supplements are taken, you will be a lot less likely to have future outbreaks.

You might also consider starting these immune tonic herbs while you have shingles. Cordyceps is believed to be effective against the shingles virus.

Energy Tonic Herbs

I have chosen several energy and immune tonics to include in this book. There are hundreds of formulas available to your acupuncturist, but they should be prescribed. The formulas I list here can be bought over the counter, and were designed to be very balanced. Which means that more people can take them with less likelihood of side effects.

Cordyceps Sinensis

Cordyceps is one of the best energy boosting herbs you can take. It strengthens your lungs, heart, and kidneys. It is a longevity tonic in Chinese medicine. It was originally a fungus that was cultured on caterpillars. It is also called caterpillar fungus. These days it is cultured on rice, and other things. I prefer this herb to Chinese ginseng. It works so fast to restore energy levels. Planetary Herbals makes a good product. It is called Cordyceps 450.

There are two main types of cordyceps. Cordyceps mycelium, and the fruiting body. The mycelium is the roots of the fungus, and the fruiting body is the most mature. There are active components in both types. The products I am listing here have been tested on patients, and we get great results in a very short amount of time.

Cordyceps Fruiting Body

Cordyceps and other mushrooms are now available as fruiting body extracts. They are much stronger if you take them as a tea. They do not taste bad. You just put a small amount in warm water, stir, and drink. You can either drink all at one time, or drink throughout the day. I have tried Freshcap Hero, and Wild Shroom. I like both of them.

Cordyceps Power CS-4

Cordyceps Power is by Planetary Herbals. It has several herbs that are strong energy and immune tonics. I often recommend it to restore health in my older patients. I even put my 82 year old dad on it. Within a few weeks he looked like a different person.

After taking Cordyceps Power for five months, his sinus and allergy problems also went away. This is a strong immune boosting formula. I have given him numerous Chinese herbal formulas over the years for allergies and sinus, but none of them worked like this. I also had him on a top quality cordyceps tablet, and he did not get these results. Allergies are caused by a weak immune system. If you take immune tonic herbs, over the long term you can treat many types of immune problems.

The herbs in this formula are Cordyceps Sinensis Mycelia, Astragalus Root, Codonopsis Root, Adenophora Root, Eucommia Bark, Eleuthero Root, Atractylodes root, and ginger root. The cordyceps is the mycelium, but it appears to be much stronger than other brands I have used. They also make a cordyceps product that has pure cordyceps in it. Astragalus is a deep immune tonic, which means that it increases the number of immune cells. Codonopsis is an energy and digestive tonic. Eucommia bark is a kidney tonic, it is also used in some blood pressure formulas. Atractylodes is an energy tonic that also reduces fluid retention. Eleuthero is Siberian Ginseng, this is a great energy tonic with less risk of the side effects of Chinese ginseng. It also boosts the adrenal glands. Ginger root is a natural anti-inflammatory, and is often used to harmonize herbal formulas.

The dosage is listed as 2 tablets. I would typically recommend two pills twice a day, at breakfast and lunch. I have seen good results with just one tablet twice a day. This formula is that good.

Reishi Mushroom Supreme

Reishi Mushroom Supreme is a mushroom blend made by Planetary Herbals. It contains Reishi Mycelia, Shiitake mushroom, Schisandra Fruit, Astragalus Root, Atractylodes, Zhu Ling Sclerotium, Eleuthero Root Extract, Ligustrum Fruit, Poria Sclerotium, Reishi Mushroom Fruiting Body Extract, Polygala Root, Ginger Root, and Cyperus Rhizome.

This product has both the mycelia and fruiting body of Reishi mushroom. Of all the supplements I researched, this one had the most evidence of healing the nerves. It is a superior herb in Chinese medicine, which means that it is one of the best to restore health.

Reishi Mushroom Supreme is a well-rounded herbal formula. It contains deep immune tonic herbs, as well as herbs that improve digestion and energy levels. I believe that taking this formula regularly will boost the immune system, and improve energy levels.

Chapter 12

How Acupuncture Relieves Shingles Pain

Acupuncture restores healthy blood flow, relaxes the muscles, and regulates nerve function. There is nothing more effective to treat any type of pain than acupuncture. LAc is the abbreviation for Licensed Acupuncturist. That is the most common title. After the LAc an acupuncturist might have MSOM, which is a Master of Science in Oriental Medicine.

In some states it is a Doctor of Acupuncture, which is DOM. In other states it is DA, or Doctor of Acupuncture. This signifies a person has a degree in Chinese medicine, which takes three to four years. If a practitioner says he or she is "certified" that might mean that the person went to a weekend class and someone gave them a certificate. You should ask your provider what type of training she has.

In addition to acupuncture techniques, Chinese herbal medicine is a big part of Chinese medicine. This will speed your healing if you are able to get herbs prescribed for you. Normally you would take a formula two to three times a day.

The reason I am explaining the licensing in different states is because it is a good idea to choose a practitioner who studied acupuncture in school for three to four years, rather than someone who took a few classes in it.

There are two common acupuncture techniques for shingles. Both of them can be effective. I have personally not found that they provide a quick resolution of the pain, but they do work for some patients.

Treatment should be given every day for the first 7 to 10 days. This is what is recommended. Herpes zoster is an intense attack on the immune system. It is more effective to get acupuncture more often in this type of situation. In China, patients get acupuncture every day. Hospital patients get acupuncture twice a day, in addition to Chinese herbal medicine.

Surrounding the Dragon

Surrounding the Dragon is when the wound or lesion is surrounded by needles. The needles are pointed toward the center of the lesion. This improves blood flow into the lesion, so the body is more able to resolve the virus. This technique is also very effective to treat scars. The scars will shrink over time. I would expect at least 5-10 treatments as a series would be needed for this to work. I did it a few times, and it did help some, but the pain came back. I believe that was because the virus was too strong, and the immune system was too weak. So this procedure might help some people. Therapy is generally given in a series of treatments.

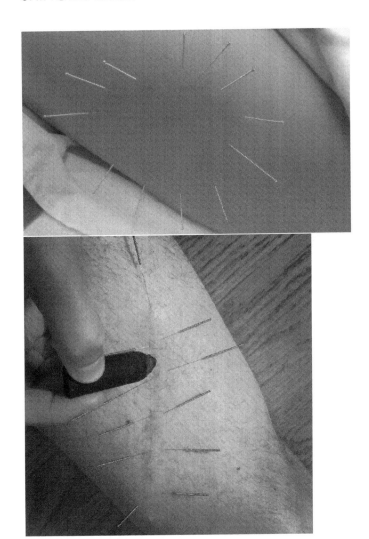

Acupuncture on the Spine

There are acupuncture points that are located a half inch from the spine. These points help to restore healthy blood flow, relax the muscles, and restore healthy nerve function. These points are located all along the spine. These points are often used to treat back pain. These points are called the Jia Ji points. It is pronounced "jaw gee." These points are famous and most acupuncturists learn them in school.

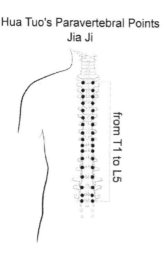

Hua Tuo's Paravertebral Points
Jia Ji

from T1 to L5

There are many other points that work very well also. A Tung acupuncture point called Ling Gu, is great for back pain. I have also found it very effective as an acupressure point. Just press very firmly into the joint by the thumb for five minutes on both hands. This point is a famous point for back pain. Any acupuncture you do to treat back pain is going to be helpful. Once the shingles lesions are gone, there might be residual back pain that needs to be treated. Please refer to the acupressure chapter for more information on this.

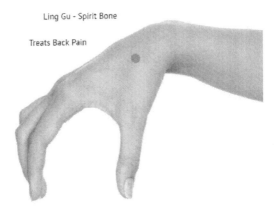

Ling Gu - Spirit Bone

Treats Back Pain

The nerves are damaged and irritated by the shingles virus. Acupuncture is always helpful to restore healthy blood flow and nerve function. I met an older woman who had shingles pain for several years. Four acupuncture sessions were all it took to stop her back pain. Any residual pain should be treated. You should expect to be pain free, and not stop until you are.

I believe it is best to purge the virus with wet cupping, then follow up with acupuncture for back pain after the virus is resolved. When the nerves are irritated, they cause the muscles to be tight. Tight muscles are the most common cause of back pain. It is very simple to treat.

Any acupuncture or acupressure treatment used to treat back pain will restore healthy blood flow in the back, and relax tight muscles. I would suggest acupuncture, because you should feel better after one treatment. Although you will probably need at least four to get the best results. Do not stop until you are pain free.

It will not benefit you to spread out your treatments. You should go twice a week. If you go more often, you will heal faster. I would also recommend the tonic herbs in the Prevent Future Shingles chapter. If you take energy tonic herbs your energy will improve, and you will heal faster and prevent future shingles attacks.

Shingles pain travels along a nerve fiber to the middle of the abdomen. It usually only affects one side, and the pain ends at the midline of the body, above the belly button. When I treat diabetic neuropathy, or nerve pain in the feet in anyone, I typically use acupuncture points on the feet, by the toes. Treating pain where the nerves end can be very effective to restore healthy nerve function.

To treat pain on the abdomen, I used points on the abdomen, where the nerve pain ended. This meridian is called the Ren meridian. I used points above the belly button. These points can also be used to treat back pain.

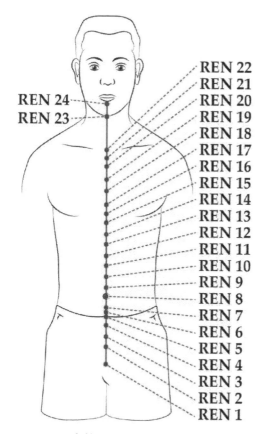

Ren Meridian - Conception Vessel

SHINGLES RELIEF

Chapter 13

Acupressure Points for Shingles

Acupressure can be used to boost your immune system and relieve pain. I will mention the points that are most likely to bring you relief.

Getting the Qi – How to Do Acupressure Effectively

There is an expression in Chinese medicine called "Getting the Qi." This means that you stimulate the acupuncture point until it is activated. With needles this is fairly easy. Although acupuncture needles are tiny, about the size of a hair, they penetrate a quarter or half inch, so they activate the points well.

To get good results with acupressure, you will need to press firmly enough, and for long enough to activate the points. If you press firmly enough, it will be slightly sore. Continue pressing for 5-10 minutes. I often alternate points. I will treat a point on one side, then switch to the other side. Both sides will work. You only need to treat one side, but it is nice to do both to balance things out and make it stronger.

The points that boost your immune system the most are Large Intestine 4 and 11, and Stomach 36. I have written a book that includes over 400 acupuncture points. It is called *Acupuncture Points Handbook*. I wrote it in easy to understand terms. It was written for patients. I compiled information from all of my acupuncture books to get the most common indications of each point.

I hope that if more people understand how each point works, they will be more likely to get acupuncture to resolve their health issues. If it is a big mystery to people, they will be less likely to get acupuncture. If you want to try acupuncture, you should always seek a Licensed Acupuncturist. This is someone who has a three to four year degree in Chinese medicine.

How to Do Acupressure

You can either use your hands to press on the points, or you can use a mini massager. I like the mini massager, because it is a stronger stimulation than using your fingers.

The massager vibrates, so the effect is much stronger than just pressing. The massager I use for acupressure comes with three different ends. I have experimented with all of these heads, and I found that the head with the most prongs on it is the most effective for acupressure.

Although I like the mini massagers, I have also had great results with just pressing on the points. It is not necessary to buy anything special to get good results.

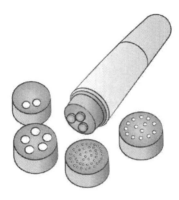

There are many brands of mini massagers. They cost about 10 dollars.

Large Intestine 4

Large Intestine 4 is also called LI 4. This point is on the hand, and it is also the number one point for headaches. It is the point you would use for any face issue, such as face pain or dental pain. It would be combined with other points for face pain, but it is great to boost your immune system. It also relieves allergy symptoms, because it boosts your immune system.

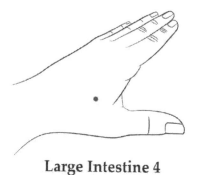

Large Intestine 4

Large Intestine 11

Large Intestine 11 is by your elbow. You do not need to be very precise when doing acupressure, as you are using your fingers to press, so it is unlikely that you will miss the point. It is located between the end of the elbow crease and the elbow bone. This point treats fevers, constipation, arm pain, and it boosts the immune system.

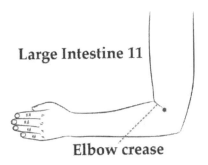

Large Intestine 11

Elbow crease

Stomach 36

Stomach 36 is the most commonly used point in acupuncture. It boosts the immune system, so it is used for colds and flu, and any immune weakness. It improves digestion, improves energy levels, treats leg pain, and treats any stomach or intestinal disorder. I have included several images of Stomach 36. You use your hand to measure down from the knee.

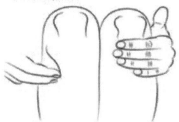

ST 36 Location

Fatigue, immune system, digestion
#1 Acupuncture Point

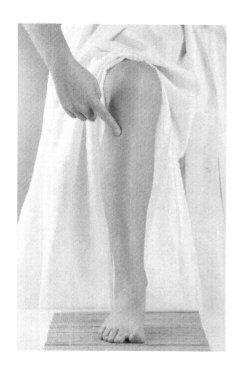

Ling Gu

Ling Gu is the Chinese name for a Tung acupuncture point. It can be translated as Spirit Bone. This point is one of the most commonly used points in the Tung acupuncture system.

Tung acupuncture is a system of acupuncture that developed over 2,000 years. This special system was kept as a family secret in China. Ling Gu is one of my favorite points treat back pain. I have also found it to be effective to press on this point for back pain relief. The most effective way to stimulate this point is to press a mini massager deeply into the thumb joint to treat most types of back pain.

I have included two images. The first one shows how close it is to the joint on the hand, between the thumb and index finger. The second image is a picture of a hand, which might make it easier for you to find the point.

Acupuncturists use line drawings of acupuncture points, because to locate most points you need to know where the bones are located. So flesh images are not very helpful for us. The bones are used as landmarks, and the points are located in the hollow area by the bones. For most points, you will feel a slight indentation when you press on the point.

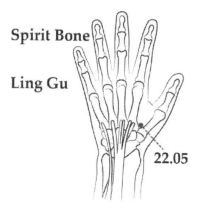

Spirit Bone

Ling Gu

22.05

Back Pain Acupuncture Treats Shingles Pain

The pain of shingles originates in the spinal nerves. So treating the back will relieve pain. The virus causes inflamed nerves, and tight muscles. This aspect of shingles is fairly easy to treat. Just treat back pain using any acupuncture points for back pain. There are over 100 acupuncture points that can be used to treat back pain.

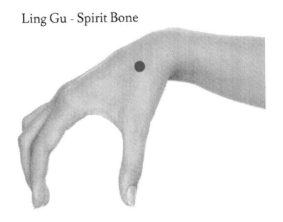

Ling Gu - Spirit Bone

Resources

The Treatment of Pain with Chinese Herbs and Acupuncture, edited by Sun Peilin

Acupuncture and Moxibustion for Herpes Zoster, Jiao, Ji-Ping, Wang, and Jun.

The Illustrated Encyclopedia of Healing Remedies by C. Norman Shealy. This book contains information on Chinese herbs, Western herbs, Ayurveda, flower essences, homeopathy, and aromatherapy.

Natural Health Encyclopedia of Herbal Medicine DK by Andrew Chevallier. Well illustrated with 550 herbs. It also includes Chinese names of herbs. This is a good reference to help in the study of Chinese herbal remedies.

Herbal Remedies, Eyewitness Companion DK by Andrew Chevallier. This is a smaller book, with 140 herbs. It is well illustrated.

Index

Other Books by Deborah Bleecker

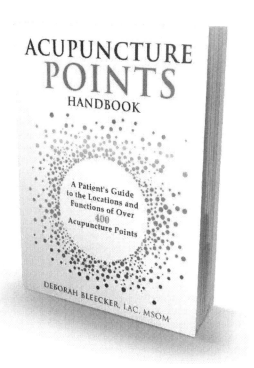

Acupuncture Points Handbook

Learn how acupuncture works by understanding how each point functions. This book was written in layperson's terms. It is easy to understand and can be used for acupressure.

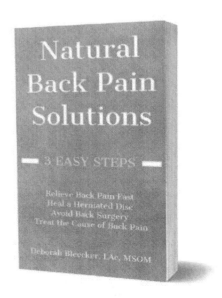

Natural Back Pain Solutions

If you take the right supplements, back pain is easy to treat.

Keep in Touch

I hope that you have benefitted from this book. So many people suffer from shingles, and there is no reason to suffer long term pain. My hope is that many people find this book and get out of pain fast. If you would like to share your story, you can contact me at deborahbleecker@gmail.com. I would like to include your story in future editions of this book.

The website www.acupunctureexplained.com is where I have placed videos and other content about this disease and others. There is also a free e-book for you if you sign up for my mailing list.

Please consider leaving a review on Amazon for this book. I would appreciate the feedback. Thank you.

23701910R00082

Made in the USA
San Bernardino, CA
29 January 2019